Foam Roller Workbook

P9-BYZ-511

Foam Roller Workbook

Illustrated Step-by-Step Guide
to Stretching, Strengthening
and Rehabilitative Techniques

DR. KARL KNOPF

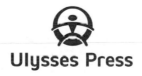

Ulysses Press

Text Copyright © 2011 Karl Knopf. Design and Concept © 2011 Ulysses Press and its licensors. Photographs copyright © 2010 Rapt Productions. All rights reserved. No part of this publication may be reproduced, stored in a retrieval system, or transmitted in any form or by any means (including but not limited to photocopying, electronic devices, digital versions, and the Internet) without the prior written permission of the publisher, nor be otherwise circulated in any form of binding or cover other than that in which it is published and without a similar condition being imposed on the subsequent purchaser.

Published in the United States by
Ulysses Press
P.O. Box 3440
Berkeley, CA 94703
www.ulyssespress.com

ISBN: 978-1-56975-925-7
Library of Congress Control Number 2011922507

Printed in Canada by Marquis Book Printing

20 19 18 17 16 15 14 13 12 11 10 9

Acquisitions: Keith Riegert and Kelly Reed
Managing editor: Claire Chun
Editor: Lily Chou
Proofreader: Lauren Harrison
Indexer: Sayre Van Young
Production: Judith Metzener, Abigail Reser
Cover design: what!design @ whatweb.com
Cover photographs: © Rapt Productions
Interior photographs: © Rapt Productions
Models: Lily Chou, Maya Craig, Lauren Harrison and Karl Knopf

Distributed by Publishers Group West

Please Note
This book has been written and published strictly for informational purposes, and in no way should be used as a substitute for actual instruction with quali-fied professionals. The author and publisher are providing you with information in this work so that you can have the knowledge and can choose, at your own risk, to act on that knowledge. The author and publisher also urge all readers to be aware of their health status and to consult health care professionals before beginning any health program.

table of contents

part 1
getting
started

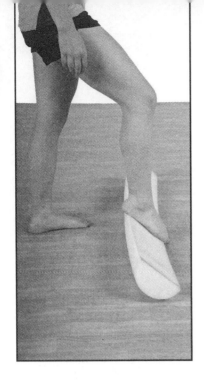

foam roller: the magic bullet?

Foam rollers were once used exclusively in physical therapy settings. In fact, Dr. Moshé Feldenkrais was credited with being the first person to use rollers for therapeutic purposes (e.g., improving body alignment, reducing muscle tightness, teaching body awareness) in the late 1950s.

Now they're used in yoga and Pilates classes to strengthen the body as well as relax and stretch tight muscles. They're also available in most gyms' stretching areas.

Some experts suggest that, if not addressed early, minor muscle imbalances (such as those tight, tender spots) can contribute to serious injuries or chronic dysfunction later on, which may require expensive therapy. Prevention is always easier and cheaper than treatment. Foam rollers are a wonderful way to address the above concerns while adding diversity and challenge to your standard exercise program.

Designing a balanced exercise routine that includes flexibility movements with strength training, cardiovascular exercise and relaxation can reduce chronic discomfort. Since foam rollers break up interwoven muscle fibers and help move oxygenated blood into those muscles, they're an excellent vehicle with which to release those tight spots in muscles (the technical term is "myofascial release") and return the muscles to a more optimal state. This can be done prior to exercising to improve range of motion, or after a workout to relax tight muscles and reduce soreness.

The beauty of the roller is that it's inexpensive and easy to use, and can be utilized to rehabilitate your body as well as prevent possible issues such as lower back pain and shin splints. *Foam Roller Workbook* provides you with numerous exercises to improve posture, core stability and flexibility, as well as hone dynamic balance and mindful relaxation.

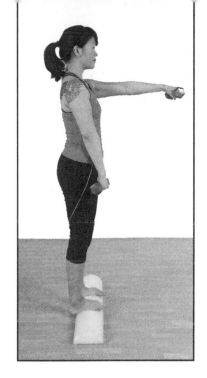

why use foam rollers?

The human body is designed in a remarkable manner and, if well maintained, will function efficiently for a very long time. Unfortunately, all too often we misuse or abuse our bodies, perhaps through activities of daily living or overuse. Whether you're highly active or sedentary, we all can benefit from a few minutes of light stretching and relaxation every day. A gentle, daily dose of movement keeps the joints lubricated and limber—motion is lotion.

More and more research in the field of exercise science shows that many of our chronic health issues can be positively influenced with corrective exercise. A former chief of orthopedics at Stanford University's School of Medicine once told me, "Modern medicine can do remarkable things, but we are nowhere close to rebuilding the human machine as well as the original equipment we were born with."

Today, therapists use progressive stretching programs and teach proper body mechanics as part of their standard arsenal to help ease clients' dysfunctions. Proper therapeutic exercise done regularly and performed prudently under the supervision of a trained therapist or personal trainer can be used to prevent injury, alleviate pain and restore your body to optimal levels.

You might already incorporate dumbbells, balance balls and resistance bands into your exercise program. Foam rollers are another tool that can provide an exciting and challenging dimension to your workout. One of the many great things about the foam roller is that it can be used by anyone, from severely disabled individuals to elite athletes. A simple adaptation can transform a basic exercise into an extreme challenge, thus allowing you to progressively ramp up the intensity of your routine and keep you from becoming bored.

A foam roller, used properly, is very effective for improving:
- Range of motion
- Core stability
- Balance
- Body awareness

- Flexibility
- Coordination
- Focus
- Body relaxation

The concept is that when you can perform an activity on a solid surface, you should progress to a less-stable platform in order to prompt your body to work harder. When you're on an unstable surface such as a foam roller, your body recruits more superficial and deep-lying muscles in order to maintain proper balance and body alignment. Some people often perform their normal exercise routine while standing or lying on a roller. By doing this, they not only isolate a particular muscle, they engage the whole kinetic chain, thus challenging all the major and deep-lying muscles.

Essentially, the exercises in this book, in concert with feedback from your health provider or massage therapist, can help you develop a better-balanced body. They'll keep your muscles toned and supple, which fosters improved functional fitness. They'll also demand that you practice proper posture and muscle alignment, which prevents joint dysfunctions and chronic pain. Joseph Pilates may have said it better: "Stretch what is tight and strengthen what is lax."

Lightweight and inexpensive, foam rollers can be stored almost anywhere, like under the bed or in a closet. Another advantage of foam roller exercises is that they can be done in the privacy of your home and you don't even need to put on exercise clothes. All you need is enough space to lie down and spread your arms.

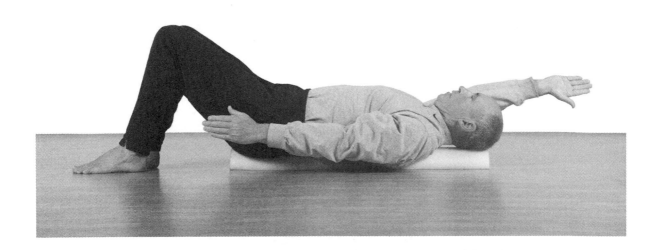

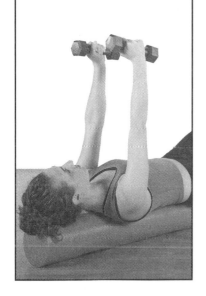

choosing a roller

Rollers come in a variety of shapes, sizes and densities and can be purchased online, at sporting goods stores and at physical therapy clinics. Selecting the type and length of roller you'll need is a personal decision, dependent on your height and weight, experience level and overall needs.

The most common roller configurations are semicircular or circular, either three feet or one foot long. Semicircular rollers, sometimes referred to as "half rollers," are flat on one side and curved on the other; they're typically three inches in diameter. Circular, or round, rollers are generally six inches in diameter.

Circular rollers are more unstable (and thus more challenging) than their semicircular counterparts. Note that you can place half rollers either flat side down or up. Having the flat side down is more stable than placing the round side down. Dense, firm rollers are good for self-massage, but if you're especially stiff, you may want to start with a softer roller so that your muscles can more easily acclimate to the pressure.

All exercises in this book utilize rollers that are three feet long, but some can be performed on shorter rollers. We refer to full-length half rollers as "FLHR" and full-length circular rollers as "FLCR."

If you're a beginner, a half roller is best. If you're looking to challenge yourself, you'll want a circular roller. Some people purchase one long roller and cut it to best meet their needs. Gyms often have various rollers you can experiment with.

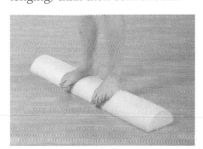 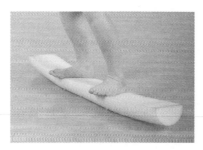 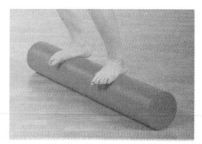

Left: Half roller, flat side down. Middle: Half roller, flat side up. Right: Circular roller.

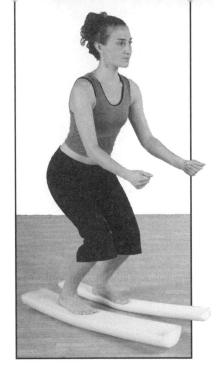

before you begin

Using a roller looks like child's play, but utilizing it correctly is no easy feat. Before you roll your way to better posture, flexibility and relaxation, you should do all you can to make sure you're performing the exercises correctly and that your exercises and massages are comfortable and things you look forward to—they shouldn't cause pain. Always tune in to your body and stop if something feels wrong. Stepping, lying, kneeling or sitting on the roller should be your time to relax, refresh and renew yourself.

Safety

Foam rollers can be used by anyone, but if you've been diagnosed with a medical condition, it's highly recommended that you obtain personalized instruction from a trained therapist prior to engaging in a roller exercise program. It is ill-advised to use the roller if you suffer from the following: severe pain, poor range of motion/flexibility, poor balance, poor coordination, and/or the inability to get up and down from the floor unassisted. It is always wise to ask your therapist to review this book and select the best exercises for you to start with. It's critical to train smart, not hard. Many of the conditions we suffer from took a long time to manifest themselves, so be patient in expecting results. Some chronic conditions such as arthritis can't be cured, but they can be managed very well with proper exercise.

Even if you're in good health, it's wise to have someone spot you when first getting started, especially when doing balance maneuvers. Also, make sure the area around you is free of obstacles. Be alert that if your muscles are tight and/or inflexible, the movements might be a little uncomfortable at first. Train—don't strain. It's better to do a little bit at first and progress slowly. Eventually, your range of motion will improve.

When performing self-massage, only use the roller on muscle—

SAFETY NOTE

Always use the roller on a firm, non-slip surface.

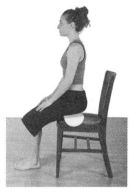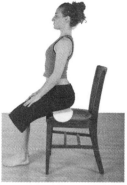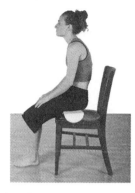

Proper sitting posture (left). Avoid overarching (middle) or slouching (right).

Lying

To lie face up on a roller (supine), start by sitting at the end of the roller. Keeping your knees bent and feet flat on the floor, slowly lie down, rolling your spine along the roller until the base of your skull rests at the other end. Use your hands as necessary for support. Maintain a normal arch in your lower back when performing all movements—do not allow your back to overarch.

To safely get off the roller, gently roll off the side of the roller onto the floor, turn onto your side, then press your hands into the floor to bring yourself to an upright position. If you're in good health and have a strong core, you can reverse the initial roll-down and come back up to sitting at the end of the roller.

To lie face up on a roller that's horizontal to you, sit on the

avoid rolling on/over joints and bony areas. Additionally, massages should be done slowly. Enjoy the experience—don't create pain. In fact, "no pain, no gain" is insane!

Getting On and Off the Roller

There are a number of ways to situate yourself on a roller: lie face down, lie face up, sit, stand, kneel. Before you can do the exercises in this book properly, you'll need to know the right way to get on and off a roller.

Sitting

Place the roller across a chair, sit on it with your "sitz bones" (the right and left tips of your pelvic bones, not your tailbone) and place your feet solidly on the floor. Your pelvis shouldn't tip forward or backward.

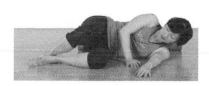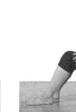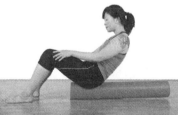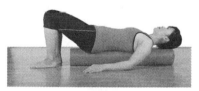

How to safely lie on a roller (supine).

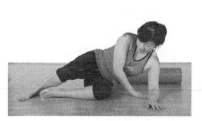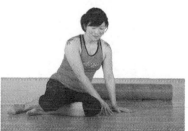

How to safely get off a roller.

floor in front of the roller and lie back on it, adjusting the roller to where it needs to be (hips, shoulders, etc.).

You can lie face down (prone) with the roller either horizontal or vertical to you. If the roller is vertical, straddle the roller in the manner of a push-up, then slowly lower your body onto the roller, aligning the roller from mid-pelvis to belly button to sternum. You can rest your head on the floor.

Kneeling

Place your knees on the roller and your hands on the floor so that you're on all fours. When

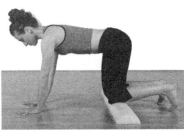

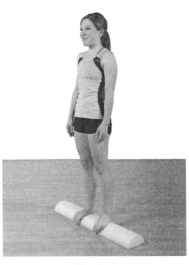

Top: Proper kneeling position. Bottom: Proper standing posture.

the exercise asks you to put your hands on the roller, just reverse the process. If the exercise asks you to kneel upright, you may want to do this next to a chair or wall for support. Keep the area clear of objects for when you lose your balance.

Standing

When standing on the roller, never compromise good posture to gain balance. Always maintain a neutral spine:

From a side view, your ears are stacked above your shoulders and your shoulders are aligned with your ankle bones.

- Keep equal weight on both feet and over the ball of your foot and heel.
- Your knees are slightly bent.
- Your pelvis should be in neutral position, neither tilted backward or forward.
- The span from your belly button to breastbone is long and lean.
- Gently pull back your shoulder blades.
- Your chin is a fist distance from your chest.

Assessment

Too often active people focus on developing stronger muscles or improving sport performance but neglect the subtle aspects of fitness, such as flexibility. Emphasizing one particular muscle group often causes that area to

become more inflexible, as well as throws the body out of alignment. Through testing, you can maximize your ability to design an effective foam roller routine.

One test checks for proper posture. Everybody wants to look younger and thinner, and having good posture is perhaps the fastest and easiest way to do both. No amount of skin lotions and potions will help if you're constantly hunched over. One of my 80-year-old students worked on her posture for a period of time. The next time she went to the doctor, the nurse took her height and said something was wrong with the measurement since my student was two inches shorter the last time. In fact, the nurse told my student that she had not been this height since she was in her 50s. The nurse asked, "People don't grow taller with age, do they?" Apparently, they can.

The other simple fitness tests check for muscle tightness and poor flexibility in two common areas so that you can focus on increasing their range of motion: the back of the leg and the shoulder region. Tight hamstrings frequently contribute to lower back pain. Poor shoulder flexibility often affects activities of daily living, such as reaching up (perhaps to get something off a high shelf) or reaching behind the back (to pull out a wallet).

POOR POSTURE

Poor posture doesn't just affect us cosmetically—it can also affect our breathing. Hunch over and try to take a deep breath, then do the same thing but while sitting or standing tall. Notice how much your ribs expand and how much air you take in.

Proper Posture: Wall Test

Stand with your heels 3 to 5 inches from a wall, then place your rear end and your back against the wall.

If your shoulder blades aren't flat against the wall, your shoulders are probably hunched forward, which can contribute to neck and shoulder pain. This is often seen in people who sit at a computer or drive for long periods of time.

If you have a significant arch in your lower back (a lordic curve), the hip flexor muscles at the tops of your thighs are possibly pulling your lower back out of alignment. You may have a greater potential for lower back pain.

If the back of your head doesn't comfortably touch the wall, you probably spend a lot of time texting or leaning too far forward, which can lead to neck pain and headaches.

If you can't place your hands on your shoulders and touch your elbows to the wall, your shoulder and chest region is too tight and can contribute to poor breathing. This is common in people, such as swimmers, who do a lot of chest work.

If your posture isn't where it should be, you can benefit from the proper posture program (page 22).

Hamstring Flexibility: Sit & Reach Test

Sit on the floor with your feet straight out in front of you. While keeping your back straight, attempt to touch your toes.

If you can't touch your toes, your hamstrings are tight and can benefit from the hamstring flexibility program (page 23).

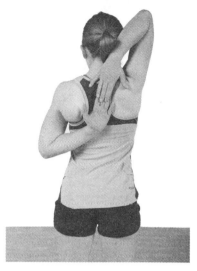

Zipper stretch test.

Shoulder Flexibility: Zipper Stretch Test

While standing or sitting, place your left hand (palm facing out) up your back and reach your right hand (palm facing body) over your right shoulder.

Can you touch your hands together? Now try it on the other side. If you can't touch your hands together, you'll benefit from the shoulder flexibility program (page 24).

part 2
the
programs

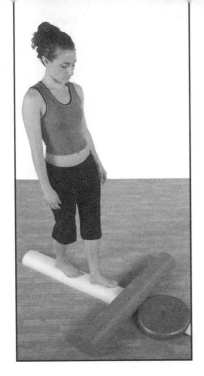

how to use this book

This section of the *Foam Roller Workbook* presents programs for a wide range of sports, including basketball, golf, swimming and running. Pick the one that best suits your needs, or use these samples as a springboard for creating your own routine. The sample routines are designed so that you start with basic moves and progress to more advanced ones. The exercises are also grouped by position on the roller as well as by categories such as stretches and massage.

The first thing you may notice when you go through one of these programs is the omission of repetitions (reps) and sets. Unfortunately, most of us are still dialed into the outdated mindset of "How many do you want me to do, Coach?" When deciding how many reps or sets of these foam roller exercises to do, the key is to forget about the number of reps you need to do and, instead, focus on maintaining proper posture and engaging the targeted muscles. You'll get better results by tuning in to your body and performing the movements with correct biomechanical form.

If that concept is too far out for you, start with 3–5 reps for active movements or 10 seconds for static positions. As the movement become easy, add more reps or think of other methods to challenge yourself. Aim to increase the number of reps to 30 or hold static poses for 30–60 seconds. Remember, more is not necessarily better. Also, when performing the movements, focus on breathing and being centered.

The exercise instructions will call for two different kinds of rollers—full-length half roller (FLHR) or full-length circular roller (FLCR). Generally, we'll start with the least challenging option (typically a FLHR with the flat side down); incorporating the FLCR is oftentimes the most challenging. However, feel free to use the one you have on hand or that's appropriate for your ability level. The FLHR is easier to control and maintain your form and balance on, but most gyms only have FLCR rollers. Be aware that it's very easy to lose proper alignment on a FLCR if you're not careful.

Designing a Foam Roller Program

Designing a foam roller program will probably be different from other exercise programs you've engaged in. To some degree, it's similar to a stretching program or even a relaxation program. You really need to listen to your body. It'll tell you which muscles are tight, how hard to press into the roller and when you've lost proper form. You need to be your own personal trainer.

When you're ready to sit down and select the exercises that should be included in your routine, consider all the movements in this book as a menu. Pick and choose according to the parts of your body that require attention. Start with 3–5 basic movements that target these areas, even if you're in great shape. Focus on doing the movements as perfectly as possible. If one of the movements is easy, find a similar exercise that is more challenging. Note that the exercises you choose may change daily. For example, if you run one day and swim the next, your body may have you do a different set of foam roller exercises each day. Just listen to your body.

The Exercises

This book features foam roller exercises from a variety of positions: seated, lying, kneeling and standing. Since one of the original uses for the roller was to provide a self-administered, deep-tissue pressure massage, often called "myofascial release," we also include a few.

The entry-level seated exercises are performed while sitting in a chair. They're designed to familiarize you with the roller and to foster improved posture and core stability.

In physical therapy or at the gym, you'll most commonly use the foam roller while lying on your back (or supine position). We also present a few exercises in which you're face down (prone).

These exercises may look simple, but they're amazingly challenging. If you're at all self-conscious, find a private space to learn them. It'll take time to be able to maintain proper alignment and stability on the roller. Think PP = perfect posture. Perfect form is more important than speed or number of reps. For this series, you may want to start with a half roller, flat side down. As you become more comfortable, flip the roller over and try the exercise from the less stable position. Once you're proficient at that stage, try a full circular roller, and once you're proficient at that, rest your feet on a pillow or any unstable surface to challenge yourself even more.

The standing exercises, all done while standing on a foam roller, are difficult and challenging. You'll want to start with a half roller flat side down. This series is best suited for people in great physical condition who also have excellent balance. Some of the movements will be done on a full-length circular roller. Since all the standing exercises necessitate a requisite level of balance, you might want to place a chair alongside you, stand in a doorframe or have someone spot you to provide support. The main focus of these standing exercises is to improve static and dynamic balance as well as core stability.

SELF-MASSAGE TIPS

With self-massage, you determine the amount of pressure you receive. However, if you've had a recent injury, consult your health care professional prior to performing any self-massages. Here are some things to consider with regards to self-massage.

- A firm, circular roller is best.
- Apply pressure only to soft body tissue, not bony areas such as joints.
- Start at the area closest to the body and roll out away from there.
- Maintain perfect posture at all times.
- Be alert to the difference between pain and discomfort.
- Don't cause pain or perform a prolonged massage on a tender area—be gentle.

The latter exercises are more advanced and include progressive resistance training designed to challenge the upper extremities. Many of these strengthening exercises can be done using an exercise band or hand-held weights.

Initially, it's useful to perform the movements in front of a mirror so that you can watch yourself, or ask a friend to observe you and kindly make corrections. If you do these moves with someone, remember that every body is unique—a movement that's easy for your flexible friend may be impossible for you.

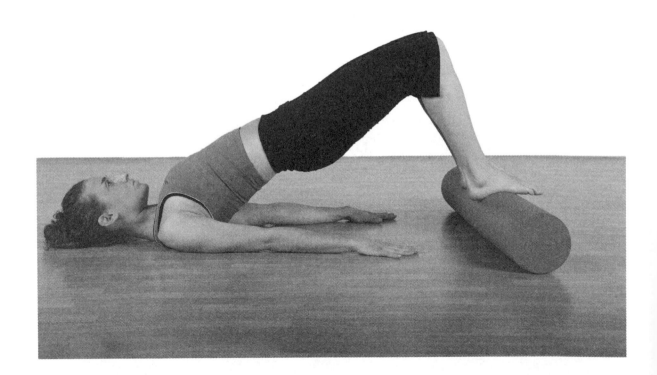

general fitness

Most healthy people who are involved in fitness programs can benefit from this general, all-over foam roller routine. It addresses common problem areas, and also covers core stabilization issues and tight muscles.

GENERAL FITNESS PROGRAM

proper posture

Too many people suffer from tight neck muscles and lower back pain, and many therapists consider poor posture to be a contributing factor. This program addresses the areas that become tight with activities of daily living and offers some movements to undo their effects. If you're unsure whether or not you'll benefit from this routine, check out the posture assessment on page 15.

PROPER POSTURE PROGRAM

PAGE	EXERCISE
40	Supine Orientation
50	Supine Fly
54	Spine Extension
78	Quad Massage
82	Hamstring Massage
79	Iliotibial Band Massage
80	Inner Thigh Massage
81	Calf Massage
86	Lat Massage
84	Upper Back Massage
48	Supine I, Y & T
51	Prone Reverse Fly

hamstring flexibility

According to some experts, the inability to touch the toes can contribute to lower back pain. Whether you're active or sedentary, you probably have tight hamstrings. This routine offers some simple methods to improve flexibility in the backs of your legs. If you're unsure whether or not you'll benefit from this routine, check out the hamstring flexibility assessment on page 15.

HAMSTRING FLEXIBILITY PROGRAM

	PAGE	EXERCISE
	77	Gluteal Massage
	81	Calf Massage
	82	Hamstring Massage
	53	Plank to Pike
	78	Quad Massage
	57	Pointer Sequence
	79	Iliotibial Band Massage
	80	Inner Thigh Massage

shoulder flexibility

For many people, rotator cuff injuries are common, maybe because we spend too much time strengthening the major muscles of the shoulder region and not stretching and strengthening the minor ones. This program helps bring balance to your shoulder complex. If you're unsure whether or not you'll benefit from this routine, check out the shoulder flexibility assessment on page 15.

SHOULDER FLEXIBILITY PROGRAM

PAGE	EXERCISE
41	Supine Stabilization—Arms
42	Supine Stabilization—Legs
43	Supine Stabilization—Combination
74	Rotator Cuff Exercise
57	Pointer Sequence
48	Supine I, Y & T
50	Supine Fly
51	Prone Reverse Fly
87	Neck Massage
86	Lat Massage

baseball/softball

Anyone who has ever played softball or baseball knows how important shoulder flexibility and core strength are. This program focuses on these often-forgotten aspects of conditioning. It would also be wise to include some hamstring and calf stretches to avoid those commonly occurring cramps.

BASEBALL/SOFTBALL PROGRAM

	PAGE	EXERCISE
	50	Supine Fly
	74	Rotator Cuff Exercise
	44	Supine Marching
	48	Supine I, Y & T
	45	Supine Pelvic Lift
	49	Supine Bench Press
	51	Prone Reverse Fly
	53	Plank to Pike
	47	Supine Leg Press-Out
	86	Lat Massage
	82	Hamstring Massage
	81	Calf Massage

basketball

Basketball is a fast-paced game that involves moving in every direction. This program helps you stretch out tight chest muscles as well as improve core strength, agility and overall flexibility.

BASKETBALL PROGRAM

PAGE	EXERCISE
50	Supine Fly
44	Supine Marching
47	Supine Leg Press-Out
56	Mad Cat
57	Pointer Sequence
58	Hip Flexor Stretch
61	Roller Squat
63	Standing Slide
70	Frontal Raise Walking Obstacle Course
84	Upper Back Massage
85	Forearm Massage

boxing/mixed martial arts

These two sports are tough on the body, which is why we include a few massages. This routine also provides exercises that keep the core hard to absorb the punishment of blows.

BOXING/MIXED MARTIAL ARTS PROGRAM

	PAGE	EXERCISE
	44	Supine Marching
	47	Supine Leg Press-Out
	52	Push-Up
	53	Plank to Pike
	54	Spine Extension
	60	Wrist Stretch
	61	Roller Squat
	62	Roller Stand
	64	Standing Mini Squat
	65	Standing Ball Pick-Up
	78	Quad Massage
	84	Upper Back Massage
	86	Lat Massage

cycling

While cycling or even casual biking is excellent cardiovascular exercise, it tends to hasten rounded shoulders and tight leg muscles. This routine focuses on stretching tight areas and strengthening the core, which is usually neglected during most cycling workouts.

CYCLING PROGRAM

	PAGE	EXERCISE
	39	Ankle Sequence
	64	Standing Mini Squat
	65	Standing Ball Pick-Up
	78	Quad Massage
	82	Hamstring Massage
	79	Iliotibial Band Massage
	80	Inner Thigh Massage
	81	Calf Massage
	56	Mad Cat
	57	Pointer Sequence
	58	Hip Flexor Stretch
	61	Roller Squat
	77	Gluteal Massage

football/rugby

You need to be prepared to play these rough-and-tumble sports, which focus on size and power. This routine strives to improve the flexibility of problem areas in order to reduce the likelihood of minor injuries.

FOOTBALL/RUGBY PROGRAM

PAGE	EXERCISE
39	Ankle Sequence
71	Lateral Raise
70	Frontal Raise
75	Obstacle Course
78	Quad Massage
82	Hamstring Massage
79	Iliotibial Band Massage
80	Inner Thigh Massage
81	Calf Massage
87	Neck Massage

golf

A common perception is that you don't need to be in shape to play golf, yet nothing is further from the truth. Your back takes a major beating when you swing the club many times per round. Unfortunately, the worse you are, the better shape you need to be in because you swing more often and walk farther. This routine focuses on core stability and basic stretching and toning.

GOLF PROGRAM

PAGE	EXERCISE
43	Supine Stabilization—Combination
50	Supine Fly
44	Supine Marching
47	Supine Leg Press-Out
56	Mad Cat
78	Quad Massage
82	Hamstring Massage
79	Iliotibial Band Massage
80	Inner Thigh Massage
81	Calf Massage
85	Forearm Massage

running/jogging/hiking

Running, jogging and hiking look relatively easy and can get you in great shape, but they can really beat up your body if you overtrain and don't stretch and massage tight muscles. This routine targets the lower extremities, tones the midsection and stretches out the rounded backs often seen in long-distance runners.

RUNNING/JOGGING/HIKING PROGRAM

	PAGE	EXERCISE
	50	Supine Fly
	44	Supine Marching
	47	Supine Leg Press-Out
	56	Mad Cat
	59	Kneel Stance
	57	Pointer Sequence
	58	Hip Flexor Stretch
	78	Quad Massage
	82	Hamstring Massage
	79	Iliotibial Band Massage
	80	Inner Thigh Massage
	81	Calf Massage
	83	Arch Rocks
	39	Ankle Sequence

rowing/kayaking

These sports put a great deal of strain on the shoulder and chest region. This routine addresses those areas by improving muscle tone and flexibility in both areas.

ROWING/KAYAKING PROGRAM

	PAGE	EXERCISE
	43	Supine Stabilization—Combination
	44	Supine Marching
	47	Supine Leg Press-Out
	48	Supine I, Y & T
	45	Supine Pelvic Lift
	49	Supine Bench Press
	51	Prone Reverse Fly
	52	Push-Up
	54	Spine Extension
	56	Mad Cat
	57	Pointer Sequence

skiing: downhill/cross-country

Skiing is a great way to spend a winter day but, unfortunately, most people don't prepare their bodies to ski. Those who do not participate in a conditioning program are at risk of injury. This routine addresses balance, leg strength and lower-limb flexibility.

SKIING PROGRAM

PAGE	EXERCISE
63	Standing Slide
64	Standing Mini Squat
65	Standing Ball Pick-Up
66	Tightrope Walk
68	One-Leg Balance
67	Rock and Roll
73	Compound Skiing
72	Skiing
82	Hamstring Massage
55	Side Salutation
77	Gluteal Massage
81	Calf Massage

swimming/surfing

Some people call swimming the perfect exercise, and anyone who has ever surfed can recall how their shoulders were tight and their lower back ached after a long day of paddling. This routine stretches out the tight muscles caused by moving your arms in the same manner over and over again. It also works on the core and balance.

SWIMMING/SURFING PROGRAM

PAGE	EXERCISE
50	Supine Fly
44	Supine Marching
51	Prone Reverse Fly
48	Supine I, Y & T
46	Pelvic Lift Marching
53	Plank to Pike
86	Lat Massage
87	Neck Massage
73	Compound Skiing
72	Skiing
76	Tightrope Challenge
69	Sword Fighter
74	Rotator Cuff Exercise

tennis/racquetball

Racquet sports are fast-paced games played on an unforgiving surface that tears up joints. This is why proper stretching and toning of specific muscles are invaluable in keeping your body ready and able to play. This routine will help you stay on the court longer and hopefully prevent injury.

TENNIS/RACQUETBALL PROGRAM

PAGE	EXERCISE
38	Pelvic Tilt
39	Ankle Sequence
50	Supine Fly
44	Supine Marching
47	Supine Leg Press-Out
48	Supine I, Y & T
51	Prone Reverse Fly
53	Plank to Pike
52	Push-Up
74	Rotator Cuff Exercise
71	Lateral Raise
70	Frontal Raise Walking Obstacle Course
78	Quad Massage
82	Hamstring Massage
79	Iliotibial Band Massage
80	Inner Thigh Massage
81	Calf Massage
86	Lat Massage

part 3
the
exercises

seated series
pelvic tilt

Goal: To improve lower back range of motion and neutral spine awareness

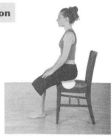

STARTING POSITION: Place a FLHR flat side up across a chair and sit upright on the roller with your "sitz bones"—not your tailbone; your feet should rest on the floor.

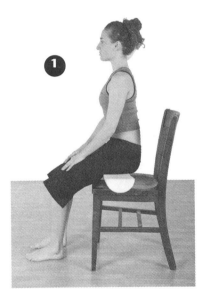

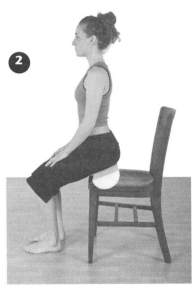

1 Slowly roll your tailbone under you.

2 Slowly roll your tailbone backward, as if sticking it out, slightly arching your back.

Continue moving forward and backward slowly, stopping along the way at positions that feel most comfortable for your back. Place that position in your muscle memory for normal activities of daily living.

VARIATION: Sit on a roller and also place your feet on a roller, flat side up, to challenge your stability even more.

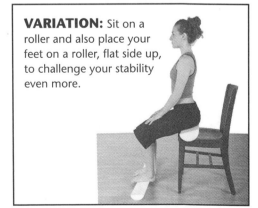

Goal: To improve neutral spine awareness and foster ankle flexibility

STARTING POSITION: Sit upright in a chair. Place a FLCR on the floor and rest your feet on top.

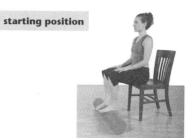

starting position

1–2 Slowly and gently roll your ankles forward and back. Remember to stay in your pain-free zone.

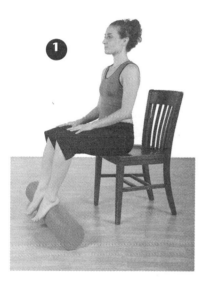

1

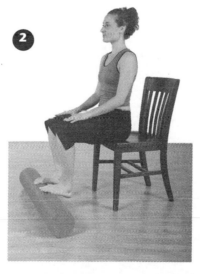

2

lying series
supine orientation

This is the starting platform for all lying exercises.

Goal: To acquaint you with the roller

STARTING POSITION: Place a roller on the floor and lie on it from head to tailbone. Place your feet on the floor, with your knees bent and arms out to the side for additional stability.

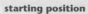
starting position

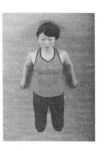

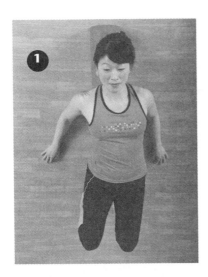

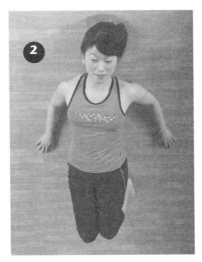

1–2 Once you feel stable, gently roll left and right and recover your balance.

3 Once you feel more stable, try lifting your arms to the ceiling while balancing in the center.

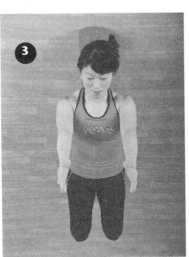

Goal: To improve trunk support

STARTING POSITION: Place a FLHR flat side down on the floor and lie on it from head to tailbone. Place your feet on the floor, with your knees bent and arms out to the side for additional stability.

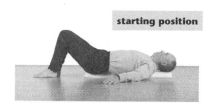

starting position

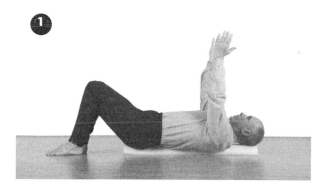

❶

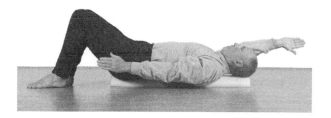

❷

1 Once stable, raise your arms directly above your chest.

2 Slowly move one arm forward and the other backward; try not to fall off the roller.

Continue alternating arms.

> **VARIATION:** Flip the roller over and perform the exercise with the flat side up, or try it on a FLCR.

Goal: To improve core strength

STARTING POSITION: Place a FLHR flat side down on the floor and lie on it from head to tailbone. Place your feet on the floor, with your knees bent and arms alongside your body. Place a tennis ball between your knees.

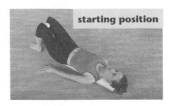
starting position

1 Keeping your knees together, extend your right leg—don't let the ball drop.

2 Lower your leg.

3 Reposition your body and perform the same movement with the other leg.

Continue switching sides, keeping your back in proper position.

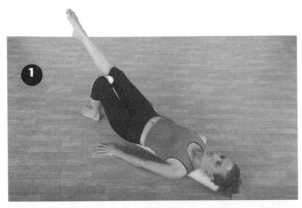

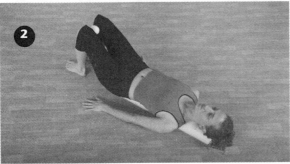

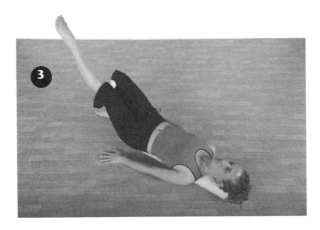

INTERMEDIATE: Flip the roller over and perform the exercise with the flat side up, or try it on a FLCR.

You can also perform the sequence with your arms lifted off the ground or resting across your chest.

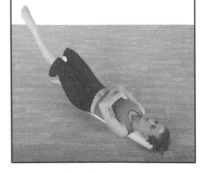

Goal: To challenge core stabilization muscles

STARTING POSITION: Place a FLHR flat side down on the floor and lie on it from head to tailbone. Place your feet on the floor, with your knees bent and squeezed together. Lift your arms up to the ceiling.

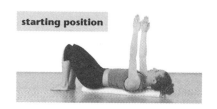
starting position

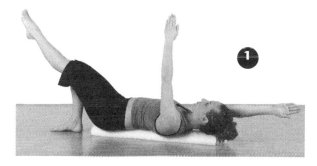

1 Keeping your knees together throughout the exercise, lower your right arm by your ear and extend your left leg.

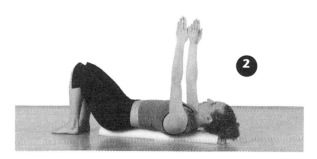

2 Return to starting position.

3 Repeat on the other side, maintaining proper form and posture.

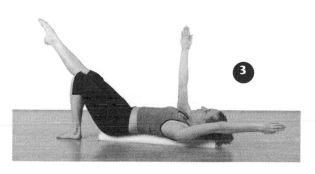

VARIATION: Flip the roller over and perform the exercise with the flat side up, or try it on a FLCR.

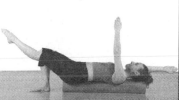

Goal: To improve trunk stability and abdominal strength

STARTING POSITION: Place a FLHR flat side down on the floor and lie on it from head to tailbone. Place your feet on the floor, with your knees bent and arms alongside your body.

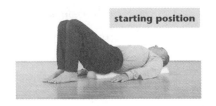

starting position

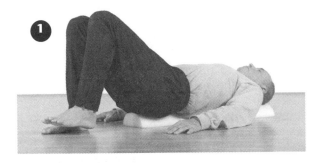

1 Once stable, slowly lift your left foot slightly off the floor (the less you lift your foot off the floor, the more challenging this exercise is). Hold this position for 5–15 seconds, making sure you maintain proper alignment. Do not allow your torso or hips to rock.

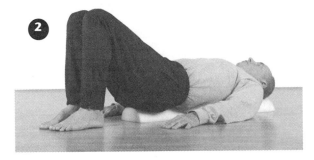

2 Return to starting position.

Switch sides.

INTERMEDIATE: Once this exercise becomes easy, try it with your arms resting across your chest or your hands reaching toward the ceiling.

ADVANCED: Flip the roller over and perform the exercise with the flat side up, or try it on a FLCR.

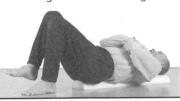

Goal: To strengthen the gluteal region, lower back and legs

CAUTION: Be careful to avoid hamstring cramps.

STARTING POSITION: Place a FLHR flat side down on the floor and lie on it from head to tailbone. Place your feet on the floor, with your knees bent and arms alongside your body.

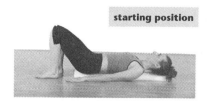

starting position

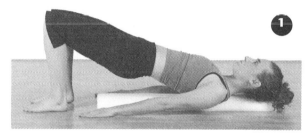

1 Slowly lift your rear end off the floor and hold for 5–30 seconds. Avoid going too high and arching your back as this can cause cramping of the hamstring muscles.

2 Lower to starting position.

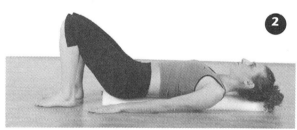

INTERMEDIATE: Flip the roller over and perform the exercise with the flat side up, or try it on a FLCR.

ADVANCED: Perform this movement with your feet on the roller instead.

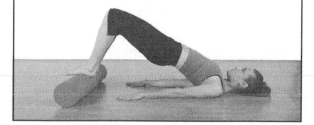

Goal: To strengthen the gluteal region, lower back and legs

CAUTION: Be careful to avoid hamstring cramps.

STARTING POSITION: Place a FLHR flat side down on the floor and lie on it from head to tailbone. Place your feet on the floor with your knees bent and arms alongside your body.

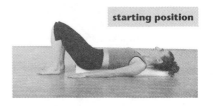
starting position

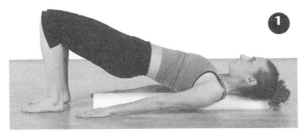

1 Slowly lift your rear end off the floor and hold. Avoid going too high and arching your back as this can cause cramping of the hamstring muscles.

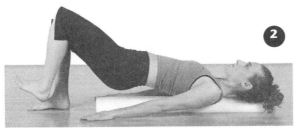

2 Once stable, slowly lift your left foot 1–2 inches off the roller and hold.

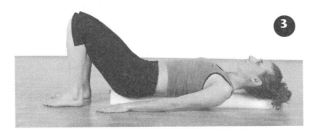

3 Relax and return to starting position.

Repeat, then switch the foot you lift.

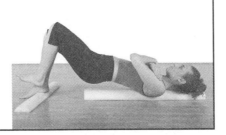

INTERMEDIATE: Flip the roller over and perform the exercise with the flat side up, or try it on a FLCR.

ADVANCED: Try this with your arms across your chest and your feet on a second roller.

Goal: To improve core stability

STARTING POSITION: Place a FLHR flat side down on the floor and lie on it from head to tailbone. Place your feet on the floor, with your knees bent and arms alongside your body.

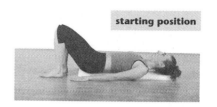

starting position

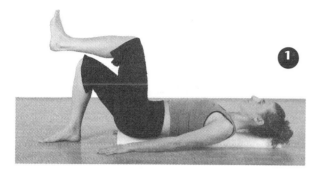

1

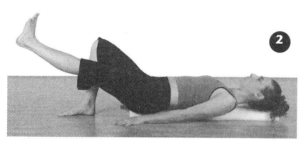

2

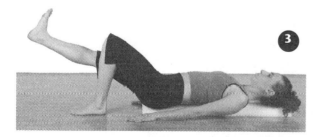

3

1 Once stable, lift your left leg so that your thigh makes a 90-degree angle with your chest. Hold.

2 Slowly press your leg forward (toward a wall) while maintaining proper position on the roller.

3 Return to starting position then switch sides.

INTERMEDIATE: Flip the roller over and perform the exercise with the flat side up, or try it on a FLCR.

ADVANCED: Start with both legs elevated to 90 degrees.

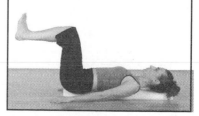

This exercise has 3 levels. Be sure to attain perfect form before moving on to the next level.

Goal: To improve core stability and shoulder flexibility

STARTING POSITION: Place a roller on the floor and lie on it from head to tailbone. Place your feet on the floor, with your knees bent and arms extended toward the ceiling, palms facing each other.

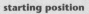
starting position

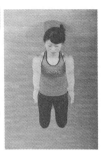

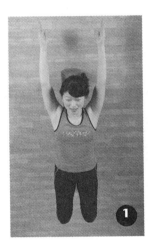

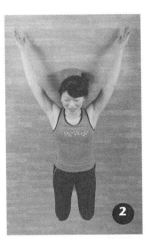

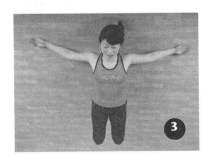

Level 1 (Is)

1 Keeping your arms straight, slowly move both arms back toward the floor, leading with your thumbs. Your body will look like an "I" from a bird's-eye view.

Return to starting position and repeat the "I" position several times before moving on to Level 2.

Level 2 (Ys)

2 Leading with your thumbs, move both arms back toward the floor and slightly out to the side in order to make a "Y."

Return to starting position and repeat the "Y" position several times before moving on to Level 3.

Level 3 (Ts)

3 Spread your arms wide apart and drop your knuckles to the floor to make a "T."

Return to starting position and repeat the "T" position several times.

MODIFICATION: If balance is an issue, try this with FLHRs, flat sides down or up.

Goal: To strengthen and tone the chest muscles (pectorals)

STARTING POSITION: Place a FLHR flat side down on the floor and place an exercise band under the roller. Lie on the roller from head to tailbone, with your feet on the floor and knees bent. Grasp an end of the band in each hand.

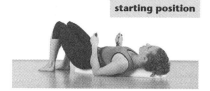

starting position

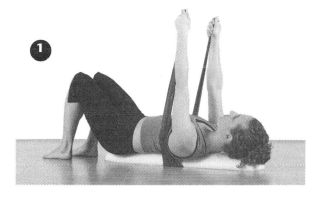

1

1 Slowly press your arms above your chest and toward the ceiling.

2 Slowly return to starting position.

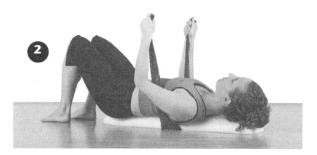

2

INTERMEDIATE: Flip the roller over and perform the exercise with the flat side up, or try it on a FLCR.

VARIATION: You can also try this with weights.

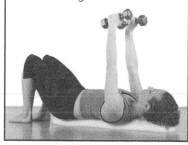

Goal: To increase shoulder girdle flexibility

CAUTION: Do not do this is exercise if you have shoulder problems.

STARTING POSITION: Place a FLHR flat side down on the floor and lie on it from head to tailbone. Place your feet on the floor, with your knees bent and arms on the floor. Once stable, reach your hands to the ceiling.

starting position

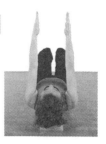

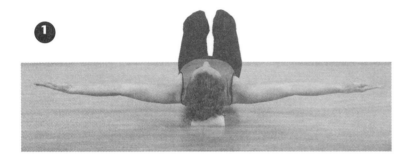

1 Slowly spread your arms out to the side; hold and relax, feeling the stretch.

2 Return your hands to starting position.

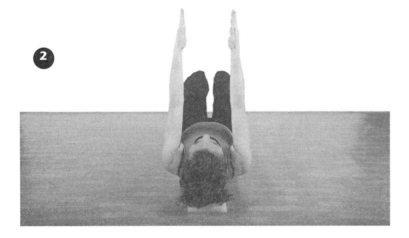

INTERMEDIATE: Flip the roller over and perform the exercise with the flat side up, or try it on a FLCR.

You can also try this exercise with weights or bands. If using a band, place the band under the roller and grasp an end of the band in each hand. Remember, trunk stabilization is the goal of this exercise, not the amount of resistance you can handle.

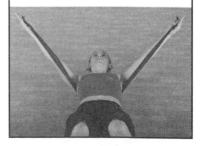

Goal: To tone upper back

STARTING POSITION: Carefully lie face down on a FLHR with its flat side up; your toes should rest on the ground. Extend your arms out to the side in a "T."

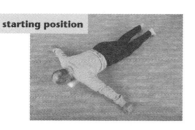
starting position

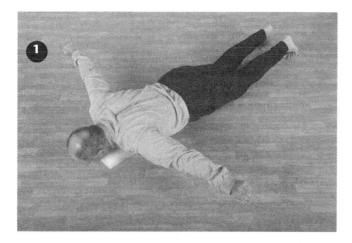
①

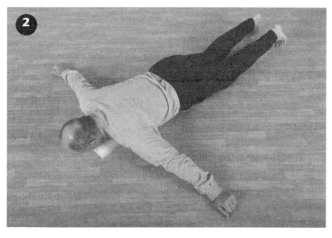
②

1 Keeping your abs tight, slowly lift your arms a few inches off the floor. Hold.

2 Return to starting position.

VARIATION: You can also try this exercise with weights.

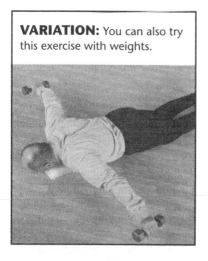

This is a very challenging exercise. Only perform as many as you can do correctly. Remember to maintain perfect posture.

Goal: To tone the upper body, chest, shoulders and triceps

STARTING POSITION: Position a FLHR flat side down under your chest, then place your hands on the roller and your knees on the floor. Once you have your balance, extend your legs behind you and assume a push-up position.

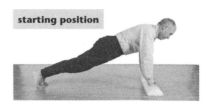

starting position

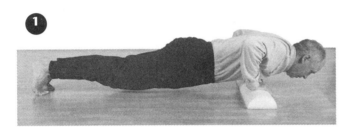

1

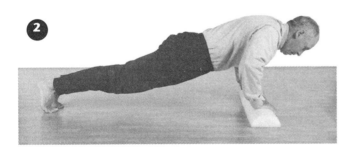

2

1 Slowly lower your chest to the roller, maintaining a straight back.

2 Return to starting position.

MODIFICATION: If you don't have the balance or strength to perform this with straight legs, try doing it from your knees.

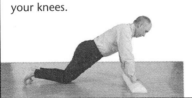

INTERMEDIATE: Place your feet on a second roller.

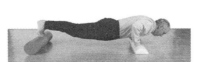

ADVANCED: Flip the roller over and perform the exercise with your hands on the flat side, or try it on a FLCR.

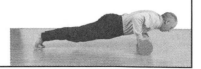

Remember to maintain perfect posture.

Goal: To tone the upper torso and improve core stability

STARTING POSITION: Place a FLHR flat side up under your toes and place your hands on the floor in a push-up position.

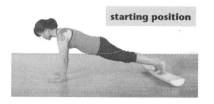
starting position

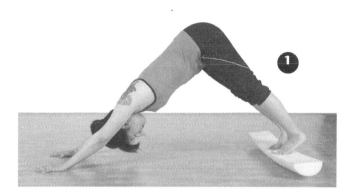
❶

1 Once stable, raise your rear end up to a pike position and hold for 5 seconds.

2 Return to starting position and hold for 5 seconds.

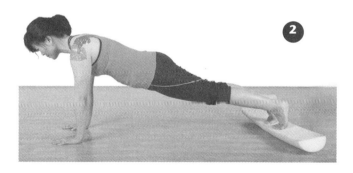
❷

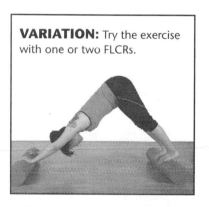
VARIATION: Try the exercise with one or two FLCRs.

54

Goal: To stretch the front of body and lengthen the spine

STARTING POSITION: Lie on your stomach with your arms extended above your head, forearms resting on a FLCR with your palms facing each other. Your legs are straight behind you and your head is slightly off the ground with eyes looking down.

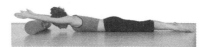

starting position

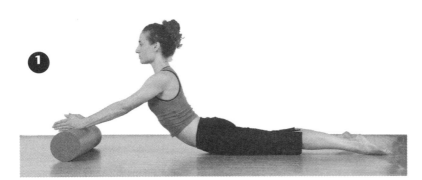

1 Slowly inhale as you roll the roller toward you, pulling your shoulder blades down. Let your head, chest and upper back rise.

2 Slowly exhale as you reverse the movement.

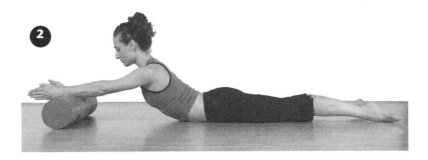

This is a very challenging exercise.

Goal: To tone the upper body and torso

STARTING POSITION: Position a FLHR flat side down under your chest, then place your hands on the roller and knees on the floor. Once you have your balance, extend your legs behind you and assume a push-up position.

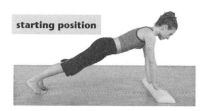
starting position

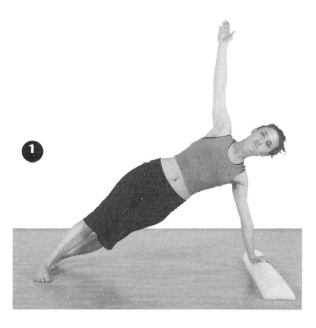

1 Slowly rotate your body to the right, relying only on your left arm to support you. If you can, extend your right arm to the ceiling so that you're in a side plank.

2 Return to starting position.

Now rotate to the other side.

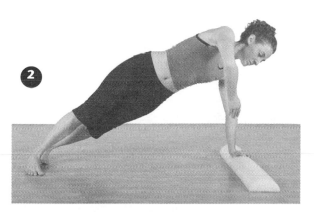

INTERMEDIATE: Each time you return to push-up position, perform 2 push-ups between rotations.

ADVANCED: Flip the roller over and perform the exercise with the flat side up, or try it on a FLCR.

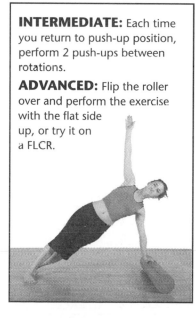

This is the foundational exercise for this series—do not progress from this exercise until you can perform it correctly.

Goal: To improve lower back flexibility

STARTING POSITION: Place a FLCR under your knees and a second one under your hands.

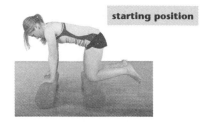

starting position

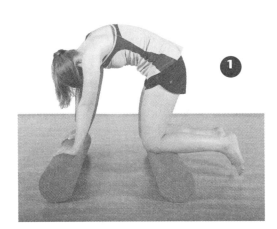

1 Inhale and pull your belly button in to round your back.

2 Exhale and slowly arch your back, letting your head rise last.

MODIFICATION: If balance is an issue, try this with FLHRs, flat sides down or up.

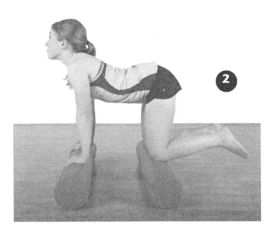

There are three options in this sequence.

Goal: To improve balance and core stability

STARTING POSITION: Place a FLCR under your knees and a second one under your hands.

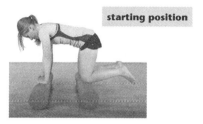

starting position

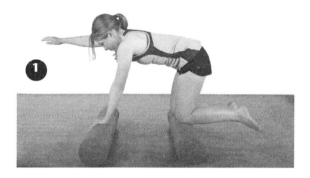

1

Level 1 (arms only)

1 Once stable and stationary, raise one arm as high as you safely can. Hold.

Switch sides and hold.

Level 2 (legs only)

2 Slowly raise one leg as high as you safely can. Hold.

Switch sides and hold.

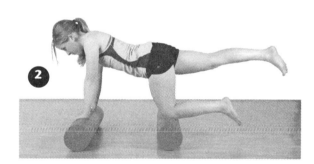

2

Level 3 (combination)

3 Slowly raise your right arm and left leg. Hold.

Switch sides and hold.

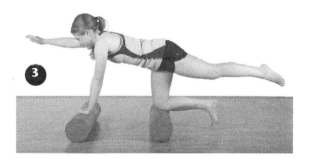

3

MODIFICATION: If balance is an issue, try this with FLHRs, flat sides down or up.

VARIATION: Place a roller under your right knee and right hand, and another roller under your left hand and left knee. Perform the series.

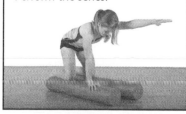

Goal: To improve hip flexor flexibility

STARTING POSITION: Place your left knee on a FLHR flat side down and your right foot on the floor in front of you. You may place your hands on the floor or have something close by to provide additional support.

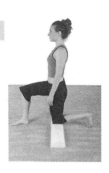

starting position

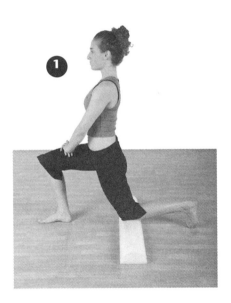

1 Slowly press your hips forward but keep your tailbone tucked in; lift your chest and keep your head high. Maintain this position for up to 30 seconds, feeling the stretch in the hip area. If you need additional stretch, slide your front foot forward.

Switch sides.

VARIATION: Flip the roller over and perform the exercise with the flat side up, or try it on a FLCR.

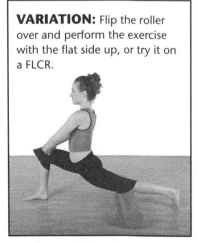

Goal: To improve posture

STARTING POSITION: Kneel on a FLHR flat side down and place both hands and feet on the floor. You may need to have something close by to provide additional support.

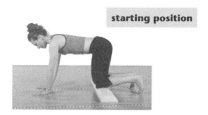
starting position

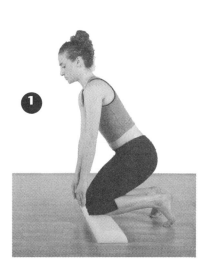

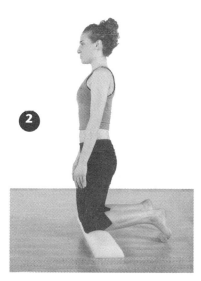

1–2 Attempt to upright yourself while balancing on your knees. Squeeze your rear end muscles and pull your belly in. Hold as long as possible, up to 1 minute.

VARIATION: Flip the roller over and perform the exercise with the flat side up. For an additional challenge, lift your toes from the floor.

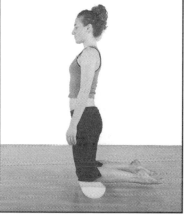

Goal: To improve wrist flexibility

STARTING POSITION: Place your hands (with fingers pointing away from your body) on a FLHR flat side up and your knees on the floor.

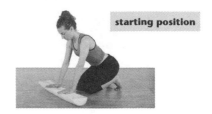

starting position

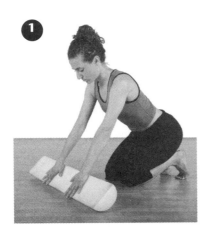

1 Slowly rock your fingers forward and hold.

2 Return to starting position, drop the heels of your hands to the floor, and hold.

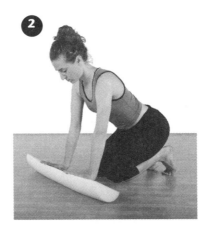

This is considered a basic foundational exercise using the roller.

Goal: To gain familiarity with the roller and improve leg strength

STARTING POSITION: Stand with your back to a wall and place a FLCR horizontally between you and the wall, around the level of your lower back.

starting position

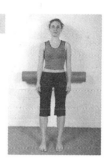

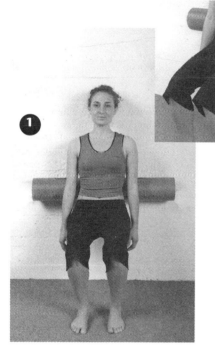

1 Slowly bend your knees to lower yourself halfway to the floor. The roller will roll up your back. Maintain body contact with the roller; the roller must remain in contact with the wall.

2 Return to standing.

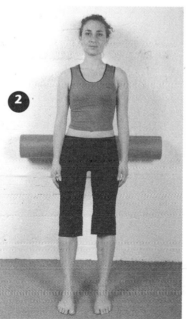

This exercise is considered one of the most basic standing moves on a roller.

Goal: To foster core stability and balance

CAUTION: If you're unable to maintain proper posture and balance, do not attempt any of the other exercises in the standing series until you can meet this minimum requirement. It's suggested that you return to the seated or kneeling exercises to improve your balance.

STARTING POSITION: Stand with a FLHR flat side down on the floor in front of you.

starting position

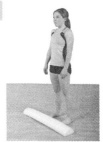

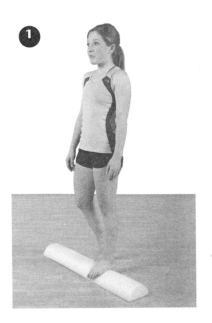

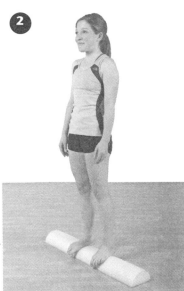

1–2 Step onto the roller with your left foot and then your right. Place your feet shoulder-width apart and maintain proper posture. Hold for 5–30 seconds.

INTERMEDIATE: Flip the roller over and perform the exercise with the flat side up, or try it on a FLCR. This is extremely challenging and should not be performed until you can do the basic exercise for at least 1 minute. BE CAREFUL!

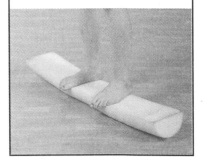

Goal: To improve balance

STARTING POSITION: Stand with a FLHR flat side down on the floor in front of you. Step onto the roller with your left foot and then your right foot; have something to hold on to for additional support if you need it.

starting position

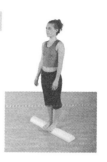

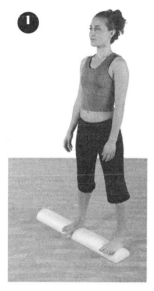

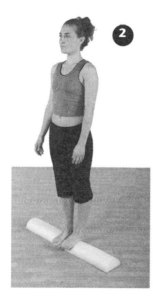

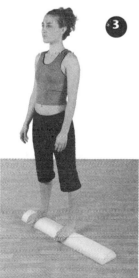

1 Slowly slide your left foot to the left and hold.

2 Slowly return your left foot to starting position and hold.

3 Slowly slide your right foot to the right and hold.

Continue sliding left and right.

INTERMEDIATE: As you advance, move your foot farther toward the end of the roller.

ADVANCED: Flip the roller over and perform the exercise with the flat side up, or try it on a FLCR. BE CAREFUL!

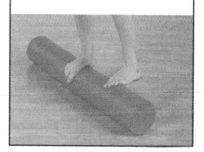

standing series
standing mini squat

Goal: To improve balance, leg strength and stamina

STARTING POSITION: Place a FLHR flat side down on the floor. Step onto the roller with your left foot and then your right.

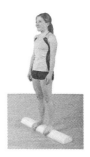
starting position

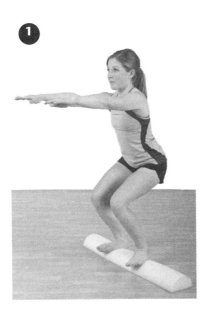
①

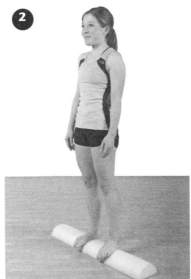
②

1 Standing in your most stable position and using your hands to counterbalance yourself, slowly perform a small squat.

2 Return to starting position.

INTERMEDIATE: As you improve, try to rely less on your arms for balance by crossing them.

ADVANCED: Flip the roller over and perform the exercise with the flat side up.

SUPER-ADVANCED: Perform the standing mini squat on a FLCR. This is extremely challenging and should not be performed until you can do the basic exercise for at least 1 minute.

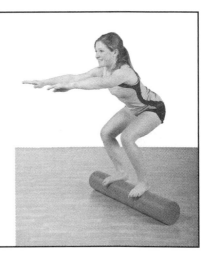

Goal: To foster better balance and core stability

STARTING POSITION: Stand with a FLHR flat side down on the floor in front of you. Place a large object such as a big balance ball or beach ball in front of it.

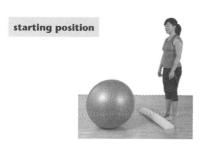

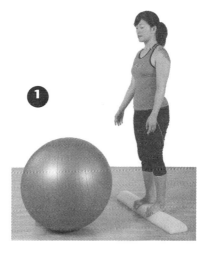

1 Step onto the roller with your left foot and then your right foot.

2 Standing in your most stable position and keeping your back as straight as possible, slowly squat down to pick up the object.

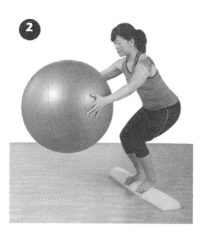

3 Return to standing.

INTERMEDIATE: Flip the roller over and perform the exercise with the flat side up.

ADVANCED: Perform the exercise on a FLCR. BE CAREFUL!

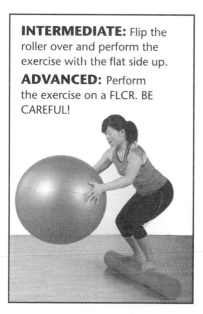

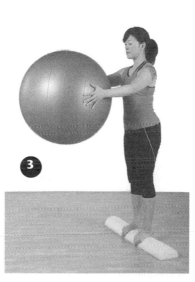

Goal: To improve dynamic balance

STARTING POSITION: Stand with a FLHR flat side down and lengthwise on the floor in front of you. You may need to place a sturdy object/chair next to you for support.

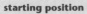
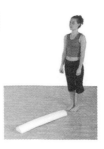

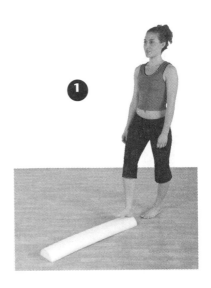

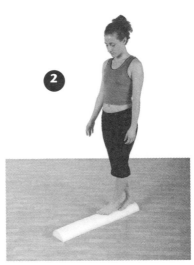

1–2 Attempt to walk the length of the roller, placing one foot in front of the other, heel to toe.

3 Step off, turn around and repeat.

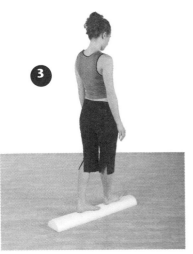

INTERMEDIATE: As you advance, attempt to walk backward or with your eyes closed.

ADVANCED: Flip the roller over and perform the exercise with the flat side up.

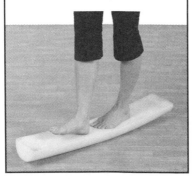

Goal: To improve dynamic balance and ankle flexibility, and to stretch the calf muscles

STARTING POSITION: Stand with a FLHR flat side up on the floor in front of you. You may need to place a sturdy object/chair next to you for support.

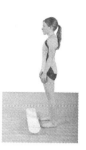

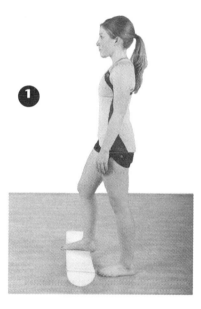

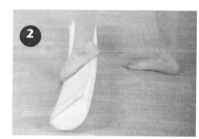

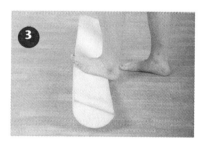

1 Place one foot on the roller.

2–3 Slowly roll your toes forward and then rock your heels back toward the floor.

Switch sides.

VARIATION: For an extra challenge, try this with both feet on the roller.

MODIFICATION: You can perform this exercise while sitting in a chair.

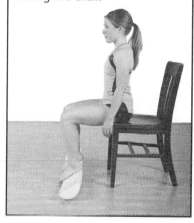

Goal: To strengthen the hip and gluteal region

This is extremely challenging and should not be performed until you can do the previous exercises in this series easily and safely.

STARTING POSITION: Place a FLHR flat side down between your feet so that you're straddling the roller. You may need to place a sturdy object/chair next to you for support.

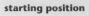
starting position

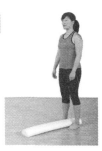

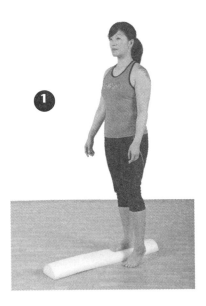
1

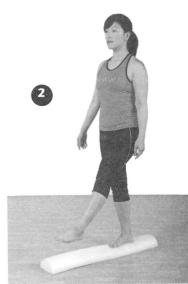
2

1 Place your right foot on the roller while allowing your left foot to provide as much stability as required.

2 While maintaining your balance, raise your left foot and stand only on your right foot for at least 15 seconds.

Switch sides.

VARIATION: For an extra challenge, try this with the flat side up.

MODIFICATION: Use a chair for support if you have balance issues.

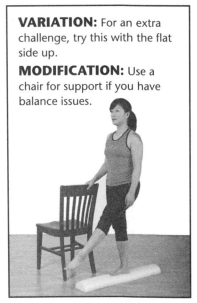

Goal: To strengthen the shoulder girdle (rear deltoids)

CAUTION: Do not do this exercise until you can safely stand on the roller for at least 30 seconds.

STARTING POSITION: Position a FLHR flat side down. Stand on it with your feet side by side and shoulder-width apart. Hold one end of an exercise band in your left hand at your left hip and then grab the other end in your right hand.

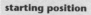

starting position

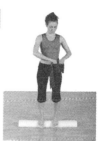

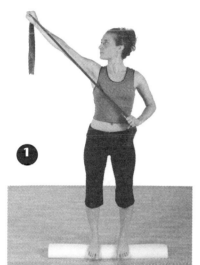

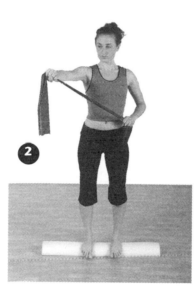

1 Maintaining your balance on the roller and keeping your left hand glued to your hip, raise your right hand diagonally across your body as if pulling a sword out of its sheath.

2 Slowly return to starting position.

Repeat and switch sides.

VARIATION: Flip the roller over and perform the exercise with the flat side up.

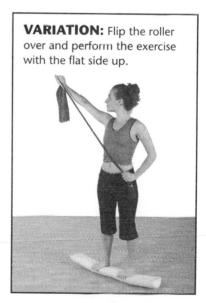

Make sure you are able to do a frontal raise correctly while standing on solid ground before progressing to this roller version.

Goal: To strengthen the shoulder region (anterior deltoids)

STARTING POSITION: Position a FLHR flat side down. Stand with your feet side by side and shoulder-width apart on the roller and hold a weight in each hand.

starting position

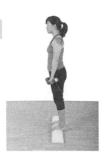

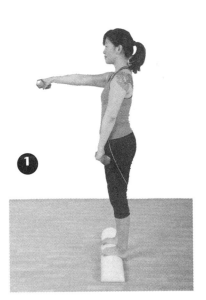

❶

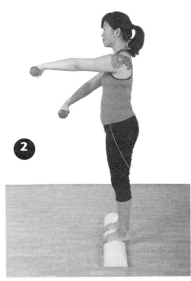

❷

1 Raise your right arm to shoulder height.

2 Lower slowly and switch arms.

VARIATION: You can also raise both arms simultaneously rather than one at a time.

INTERMEDIATE: Flip the roller over and perform the exercise with the flat side up.

You can also stand on the roller with one foot in front of the other and perform the movement, then place the other foot in front.

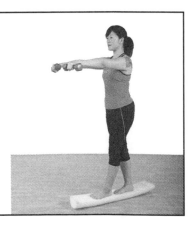

Make sure you are able to do a lateral raise correctly while standing on solid ground before progressing to this roller version.

Goal: To strengthen the shoulder region (lateral deltoids)

STARTING POSITION: Position a FLHR flat side down. Stand on it with your feet side by side and shoulder-width apart. Hold a weight in each hand.

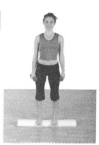

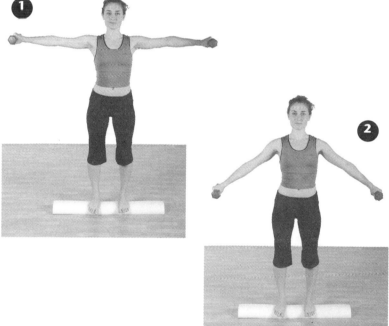

1 Raise your hands out to the side, stopping at shoulder height.

2 Lower slowly.

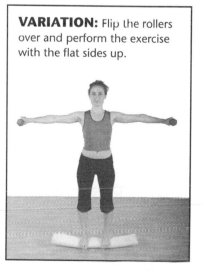

VARIATION: Flip the rollers over and perform the exercise with the flat sides up.

Goal: To learn to distribute your weight evenly

STARTING POSITION: Stand with two FLHRs side by side (shoulder-width apart) on the floor, flat sides down. You may need to place a sturdy object/chair next to you for support.

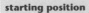

starting position

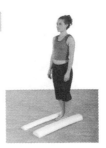

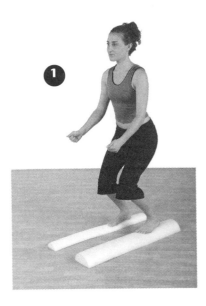

1 Place one foot on one roller and the other foot on the other roller, as if skiing. Maintain balance and proper posture and hold.

INTERMEDIATE: As you advance, slowly shift your weight from one side to the other and hold for 30–60 seconds.

You can also try it with your eyes closed.

ADVANCED: Flip the rollers over and perform the exercise with the flat sides up.

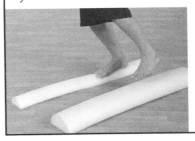

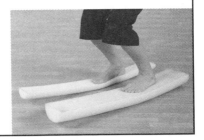

Goal: To learn to distribute your weight evenly while performing strength and conditioning exercises

STARTING POSITION: Stand with two FLHRs side by side (shoulder-width apart) on the floor, flat sides down. You may need to place a sturdy object/chair next to you for support. Place one foot on one roller and the other foot on the other roller, as if skiing.

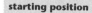

starting position

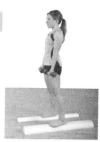

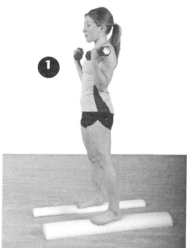

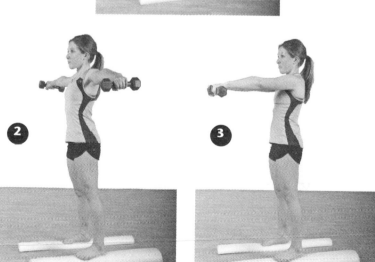

1 Maintain balance and proper posture as you perform arm curls (with or without light handweights).

2 Perform lateral raises (with or without light handweights).

3 Perform frontal raises (with or without light handweights).

VARIATION: Flip the rollers over and perform the motions with the flat sides up.

Make sure you are able to do this exercise correctly while standing on solid ground before progressing to this roller version.

Goal: To strengthen the shoulder complex

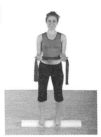

STARTING POSITION: Position a FLHR flat side down. Stand on it with your feet side by side and shoulder-width apart. Grasp an end of an exercise band in each hand in front of your body. Bend your elbows 90 degrees and keep your elbows by your ribs.

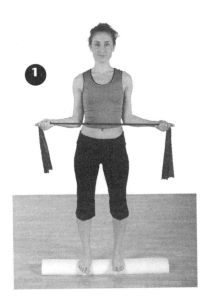

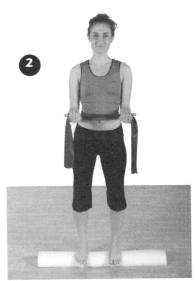

1 With your elbows glued to your ribs, slowly swing your hands comfortably out to the side.

2 Return to starting position.

VARIATION: Flip the roller over and perform the exercise with the flat side up.

MODIFICATION: Rather than swinging both hands out at once, do one hand at a time.

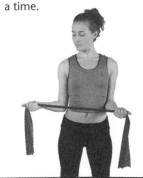

This advanced exercise should not be performed by anyone who is not extremely stable on their feet.

Goal: To improve dynamic balance, agility and coordination

STARTING POSITION: Scatter different-sized rollers in a small area. If possible, the rollers should have different densities. Place some flat side up, others rounded side up. Be creative in the design of your course. Start easy and progressively challenge yourself.

starting position

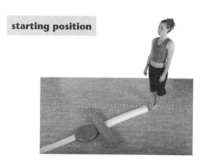

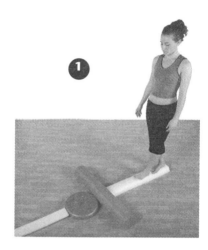

1–2 Carefully step over or cross a roller, pausing momentarily and maintaining your balance.

3 Continue performing this course.

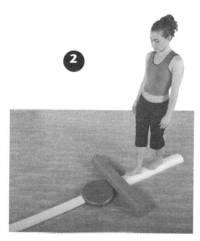

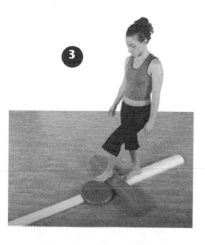

VARIATION: Once you're proficient at this, try to stop and pick up an object while standing on one leg. Be creative in thinking of ways to challenge your balance.

This advanced exercise should not be performed by anyone who is not extremely stable on their feet.

Goal: To improve dynamic and static balance

STARTING POSITION: Line up several FLHRs of various heights and densities in a line, with some flat sides up and others flat sides down.

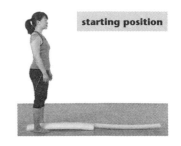

starting position

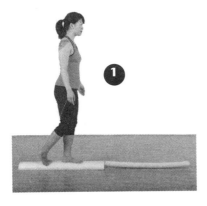

1

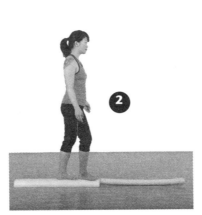

2

1–3 Carefully walk on top of the rollers, doing your best not to fall off.

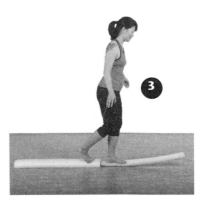

3

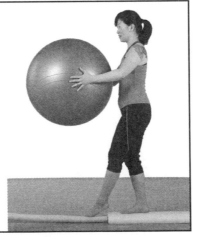

INTERMEDIATE: As you progress, rather than having your hands and arms out to the side, try to maintain your balance with your arms alongside your body or while holding a ball.

ADVANCED: Once you're proficient at this, try walking while holding a tray of marbles.

Goal: To improve circulation and release tight gluteal muscles

STARTING POSITION: Sit on a FLCR that's either placed horizontally on the floor or a chair. Shift your weight so that you're on one butt cheek.

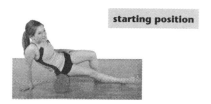

starting position

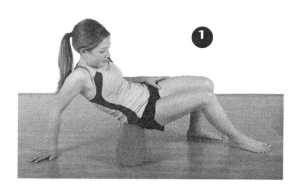

①

1–2 Slowly roll your rear end forward then backward, stopping at any point along the way that requires a little more attention. You can also slowly lean to the left and hold, and then shift your weight to the right.

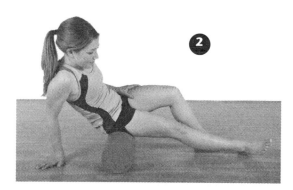

②

Goal: To relieve tight thigh muscles

STARTING POSITION: Lie face down and place a FLCR under your thighs. Place your hands on the floor for support.

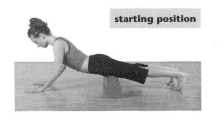
starting position

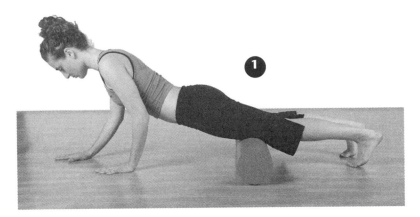

1 Slowly roll the roller down toward the knee area. Do not roll on or over the knees.

2 Slowly roll the roller back up toward your hips, stopping at spots along the way that require more attention.

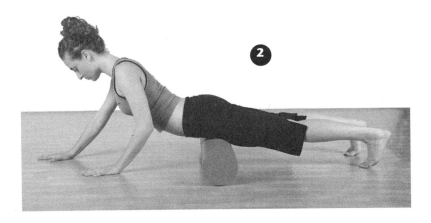

Goal: To massage the IT band/upper-outer thigh

STARTING POSITION: Lie on one side and place a FLCR under your bottom leg. Use your hands and other foot for support.

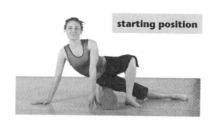

starting position

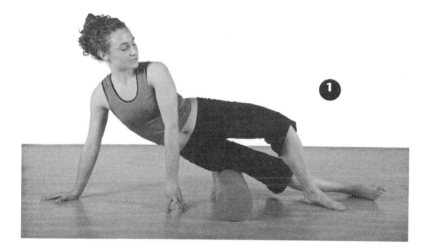

1

1 Starting just below the hip bone, slowly roll the roller toward, but stop just above, the knee.

2 Slowly roll the roller back up toward the hip, stopping at spots along the way that require more attention.

Switch sides.

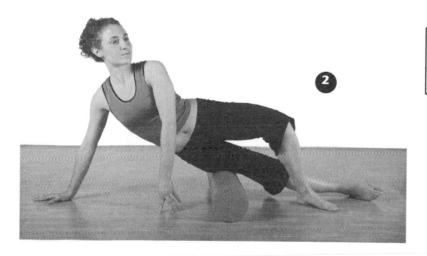

2

VARIATION: You can also pause at a tight spot and rock from side to side.

Goal: To massage the inner leg

STARTING POSITION: Lie on one side and place a FLCR between your thighs. You can keep your leg straight or slightly bent.

starting position

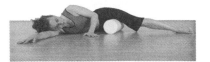

1 Slowly and gently roll your top leg up and down the roller. Along the way, stop and apply gentle pressure wherever additional attention is needed.

Switch sides.

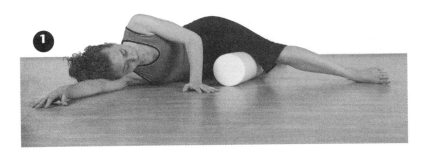

VARIATION: While lying on your side, you can also place the roller between your thighs and let gravity do the work.

Goal: To massage the calf muscle

STARTING POSITION: Sit on the floor with one knee bent and the other leg straight. Place a FLCR horizontally beneath the calf muscle of the straight leg.

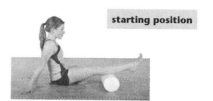

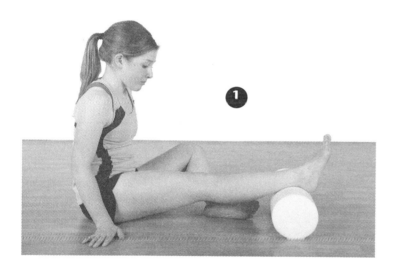

1 Slowly roll the roller up and down the leg, between the knee and ankle. Along the way, stop wherever additional attention is needed and press down to generate just enough pressure to release the tension.

Switch sides.

VARIATION: You can also place both legs on the roller and lift your rear end off the floor by supporting yourself with your hands.

massage series
hamstring massage

Goal: To massage the back of the thigh

STARTING POSITION: Sit on the floor with one knee bent and the other leg straight. Place a FLCR horizontally beneath the hamstring of your straight leg.

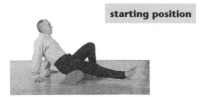

starting position

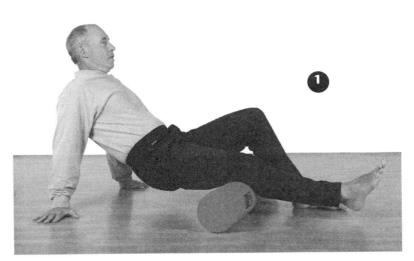

1 Slowly roll the leg up and down the roller. Along the way, stop wherever additional attention is needed and apply just enough pressure to release tension.

Switch sides.

VARIATION: You can also straighten both legs and roll them up and down the roller.

Goal: To massage the arches of your feet

STARTING POSITION: Sit in a chair and place both feet in the middle of a FLCR.

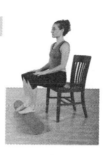

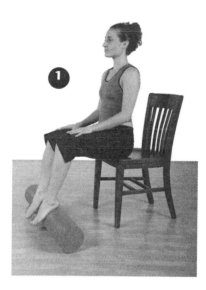

1–2 Slowly roll your feet forward and then backward to massage the arches and bottoms of your feet. Along the way, stop and apply additional pressure where needed.

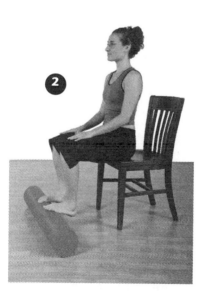

Goal: To open up the chest region and relax the upper back muscles

STARTING POSITION: Place a FLCR on the floor and lie on it horizontally from shoulder to shoulder, just beneath your shoulder blades. Place your feet on the floor, with your knees bent and hands lightly clasped behind your head. Keep your elbows wide.

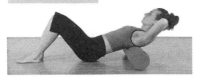

starting position

1 Gently roll toward your upper shoulders and then your lower shoulder blades, stopping to apply additional pressure where needed.

> **VARIATION:** You can also do this by lying on the roller from head to tailbone and gently rolling from left to right.

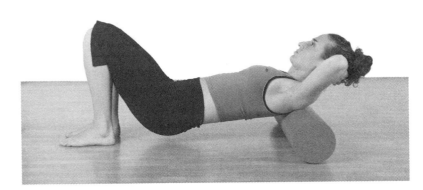

Goal: To massage the inner part of the forearm

STARTING POSITION: Kneel in front of a FLCR and place your forearms on the roller with your palms face down.

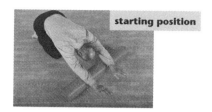
starting position

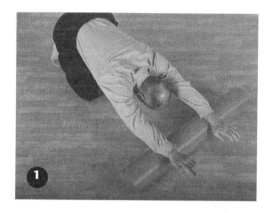

1–2 Slowly move your arms forward and back. Along the way, stop and apply pressure wherever additional attention is needed.

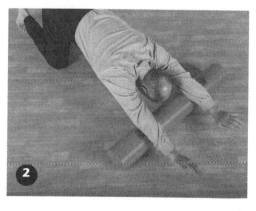

Goal: To massage the latissimus dorsi

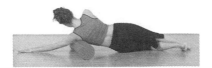

starting position

STARTING POSITION: Lie on your left side and extend your left arm straight up along the floor. Place a FLCR just below your armpit.

❶

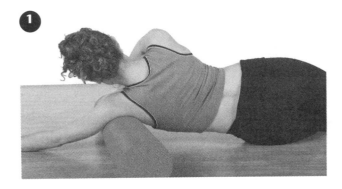

❷

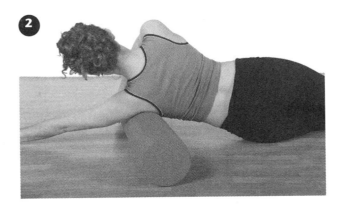

1–2 Slowly roll your body up and down along the roller. Along the way, stop and apply pressure wherever additional attention is needed.

Switch sides.

VARIATION: You can also pause at a tight spot and rock from side to side.

Goal: To relax and stretch the neck and upper shoulder region

STARTING POSITION: Lie on your back with your knees bent, feet on the floor and arms along your sides. Position a FLCR under the base of your head. Slowly breathe in through your nose and out through your mouth as you allow your back to settle and relax.

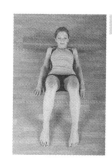

starting position

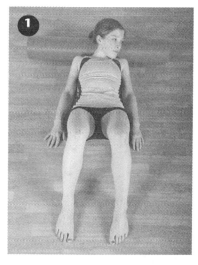

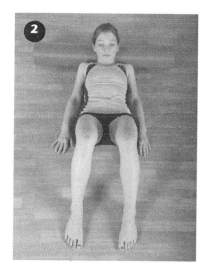

1 Inhale as you gently and slowly look to the left.

2 Exhale as you return to starting position.

3 Inhale as you look to the right.

4 Exhale as you return to starting position.

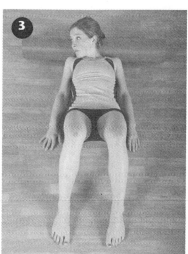

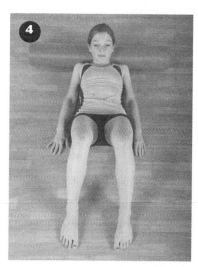

index

other books by karl knopf

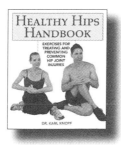

Healthy Hips Handbook
$14.95
Healthy Hips Handbook is designed to help prevent hip problems for some and, for those with existing hip problems, provide post-rehabilitation exercises.

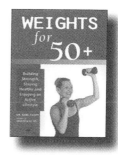

Weights for 50+
$14.95
Weight training is one of the most effective ways to get healthy and fight the physical signs of aging. *Weights for 50+* shows how easy it is for anyone to get started with weights.

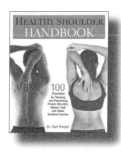

Healthy Shoulder Handbook
$15.95
Includes an overview of shoulder anatomy so anyone can use this friendly manual to strengthen an injured shoulder, identify the onset of a shoulder problem, or better understand injury prevention.

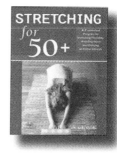

Stretching for 50+
$14.95
Based on the belief that individuals over 50 can do most of the same things as 20- and 30-year-olds, this book shows how to maintain and improve flexibility by incorporating stretching into one's life.

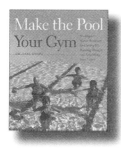

Make the Pool Your Gym
$14.95
Shows how to create an effective and efficient water workout that can build strength, improve cardiovascular fitness, and burn calories.

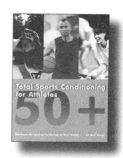

Total Sports Conditioning for Athletes 50+
$14.95
Provides sport-specific workouts that allow aging athletes to maintain the flexibility, strength, and speed needed to win.

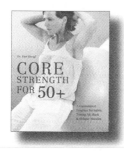

Core Strength for 50+
$15.95
Core Strength for 50+ provides more than 75 exercises that build and maintain strong muscles in the abs, obliques, lower back and butt.

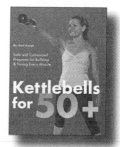

Kettlebells for 50+
$14.95
Offers progressive programs that will improve strength, foster core stability, increase hand-eye coordination, boost mind-body awareness, and enhance sports performance.

To order these books call 800-377-2542 or 510-601-8301, fax 510-601-8307, e-mail ulysses@ulyssespress.com, or write to Ulysses Press, P.O. Box 3440, Berkeley, CA 94703. All retail orders are shipped free of charge. California residents must include sales tax. Allow two to three weeks for delivery.

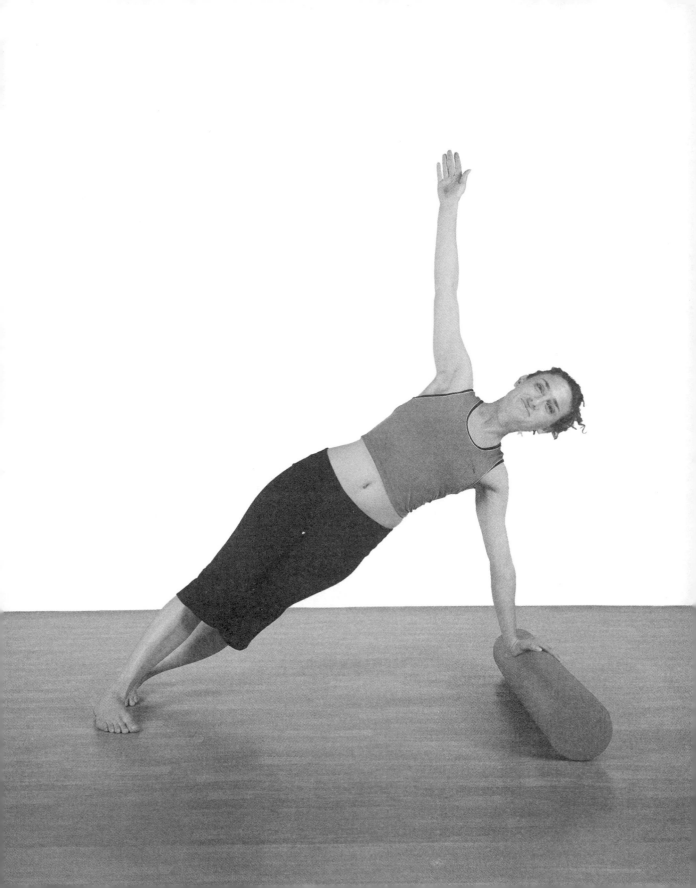

acknowledgments

It is a joy to work with such a team of professionals, without whose skill and expertise this book would not have been possible. I would like to sincerely thank Lily Chou and Claire Chun, whose attention to detail and ability to explain complex concepts in user-friendly terms is without parallel. Thanks also to models Lily Chou, Maya Craig and Lauren Harrison for their patience, and to Austin Forbord and his team at Rapt Productions, who were able to capture the essence of the exercises so well. I'd like to thank acquisitions editors Keith Riegert and Kelly Reed for their vision. Lastly, a special note of appreciation to my son Chris Knopf, who served as my fact checker. Special thanks to my wife Margaret of 30-plus years for so graciously allowing me private time in the living room to write this and other books.

about the author

KARL KNOPF, author of *Healthy Hips Handbook*, *Healthy Shoulder Handbook*, *Stretching for 50+*, *Weights for 50+* and *Total Sports Conditioning for Athletes 50+*, has been involved with the health and fitness of the disabled and older adults for 30 years. A consultant on numerous National Institutes of Health grants, Knopf has served as advisor to the PBS exercise series *Sit and Be Fit*, and to the State of California on disabilities issues. He is a frequent speaker at conferences and has written several textbooks and articles. Knopf coordinates the Fitness Therapist Program at Foothill College in Los Altos Hills, California.